UNLEASHING YOUR INNER CALM

Strategies for Regulating Your Nervous System and Reducing Stress

John Stott

Table of Contents

CHAPTER 1: UNDERSTANDING THE NERVOUS SYSTEM

- **Brief overview of the anatomy and function of the nervous system**

The nervous system is a complex network of cells and tissues that control and coordinate the functions of the body. It is divided into two main parts: the central nervous system (CNS) and the peripheral nervous system (PNS).

1. Central Nervous System (CNS): The CNS is composed of the brain and spinal cord. The brain is responsible for receiving and interpreting sensory information, generating thoughts and emotions, and coordinating movement and behavior. The spinal cord is a long, thin bundle of nerves that connects the brain to the rest of the body and acts as a relay center for incoming and outgoing signals.

2. Peripheral Nervous System (PNS): The PNS is composed of all the nerves that lie outside of the CNS and connect it to the rest of the body. It is divided into two main parts: the somatic nervous system and the autonomic nervous system.

a. Somatic Nervous System: The somatic nervous system controls voluntary movement and sensation in the body, such as touch and temperature.

b. Autonomic Nervous System: The autonomic nervous system controls automatic functions such as heart rate, digestion, and breathing. It is further divided into two parts: the sympathetic nervous system and the parasympathetic nervous system. The sympathetic nervous system prepares the body for fight or flight responses in times of stress, while the parasympathetic nervous system works to calm the body and promote relaxation.

The nervous system functions by transmitting signals or electrical impulses along nerve fibers called axons. These signals are transmitted from one neuron to another across synapses, specialized structures that allow communication between neurons. The nervous system plays a critical role in maintaining homeostasis, or balance, in the body, and any malfunction or damage can have significant impacts on physical and mental health.

- **The role of the autonomic nervous system in regulating automatic bodily functions**

The autonomic nervous system (ANS) is responsible for regulating automatic bodily functions such as heart rate, digestion, breathing, and other internal processes. It is comprised of two branches: the sympathetic nervous system and the parasympathetic nervous system, which work in opposition to maintain balance in the body.

1. Sympathetic Nervous System: The sympathetic nervous system is responsible for the body's "fight or flight" response. When activated, it increases heart rate, blood pressure, and respiration, and diverts blood flow to the muscles and away from the digestive system. This helps prepare the body for physical exertion and heightened alertness in times of stress or danger.

2. Parasympathetic Nervous System: The parasympathetic nervous system counteracts the effects of the sympathetic nervous system and is responsible for the "rest and digest" response. When activated, it slows heart rate, lowers blood pressure, and increases blood flow to the digestive system. This helps calm the body and promote relaxation.

The autonomic nervous system works to maintain a balance between the sympathetic and parasympathetic responses and to regulate a wide range of automatic bodily functions. This includes functions such as regulating blood pressure, controlling breathing, managing the production of hormones, and controlling the function of the digestive, urinary, and reproductive systems.

Abnormalities or imbalances in the autonomic nervous system can result in various health conditions, such as high blood pressure, heart disease, digestive problems, and sexual dysfunction. To maintain optimal health, it is important to engage in activities and habits that promote a balanced and healthy autonomic nervous system, such as exercise, stress management, and a healthy diet.

CHAPTER 2: PRACTICING RELAXATION TECHNIQUES

- Deep breathing exercises

Deep breathing exercises are a type of breathing technique that involves inhaling and exhaling deeply and slowly. These exercises are used for a variety of purposes, including reducing stress and anxiety, improving relaxation, and boosting overall physical and mental well-being.

1. How to practice: To perform deep breathing exercises, find a quiet and comfortable place to sit or lie down. Begin by breathing in slowly and deeply through your nose, filling your lungs completely. Hold your breath for a few seconds, then exhale slowly through your mouth. Repeat this pattern several times, inhaling deeply and exhaling slowly, focusing on your breath and trying to calm your mind.

2. Benefits: Deep breathing exercises have been shown to have several health benefits, including:

a. Reduced stress and anxiety: By slowing down breathing, deep breathing exercises help to activate the body's relaxation response and reduce stress and anxiety levels.

b. Improved sleep: Regular deep breathing exercises can help promote better sleep by reducing feelings of stress and tension.

c. Improved respiratory function: By expanding the lungs and strengthening the muscles used in breathing, deep breathing exercises can improve respiratory function and lung capacity.

d. Enhanced immune function: Deep breathing exercises have been shown to improve the function of the immune system by increasing the flow of oxygen to the body's tissues.

3. Precautions: Deep breathing exercises are generally safe for most people, but it is important to check with a doctor before starting if you have any health conditions that affect breathing. Additionally,

people with certain conditions, such as panic disorder or hyperventilation syndrome, may experience symptoms such as lightheadedness, dizziness, or chest pain during deep breathing exercises. If this occurs, it is important to stop and seek medical advice.

Overall, deep breathing exercises are a simple and effective way to promote relaxation and improve overall health and well-being. Regular practice can help to reduce stress and anxiety, improve sleep, and enhance respiratory function.

- Progressive muscle relaxation

Progressive muscle relaxation (PMR) is a stress management technique that involves tensing and relaxing different muscle groups in a specific order. The goal of PMR is to reduce physical tension and promote feelings of relaxation and calm.

1. How to practice: To perform PMR, find a quiet and comfortable place to sit or lie down. Begin by tensing a specific muscle group, such as your fists or feet, for several seconds. Then, slowly release the tension and focus on the feeling of relaxation in the muscles. Move through different muscle groups, tensing and relaxing each one in turn, and pay attention to the sensations of tension and relaxation in each area.

2. Benefits: PMR has been shown to have several health benefits, including:

a. Reduced stress and anxiety: By reducing physical tension, PMR can help to activate the body's relaxation response and reduce stress and anxiety levels.

b. Improved sleep: PMR can help promote better sleep by reducing feelings of stress and tension and promoting relaxation.

c. Improved physical functioning: By reducing muscle tension, PMR can improve overall physical functioning and reduce the risk of physical problems such as headaches, neck and back pain, and muscle cramps.

d. Enhanced mental clarity: By promoting relaxation and reducing physical tension, PMR can improve mental clarity and increase feelings of calm and focus.

3. Precautions: PMR is generally safe for most people, but it is important to check with a doctor before starting if you have any health conditions that affect muscle function or mobility. Additionally, PMR may not be suitable for individuals with certain mental health conditions, such as anxiety disorders or depression. If you experience any discomfort or pain during PMR, it is important to stop and seek medical advice.

Overall, PMR is a simple and effective technique for reducing stress and promoting relaxation. Regular practice can help to reduce physical tension, improve sleep, and enhance overall well-being.

- Meditation and mindfulness

Meditation and mindfulness are practices that focus on bringing awareness and attention to the present moment. They are often used as stress-management techniques and to promote physical and mental well-being.

1. Meditation: Meditation is a practice that involves focusing the mind on a specific object, sound, movement, or the breath. The goal of meditation is to quiet the mind and promote a state of relaxation and inner calm. There are many different forms of meditation, including mindfulness meditation, guided meditation, and movement meditation.

2. Mindfulness: Mindfulness is a specific form of meditation that involves paying attention to the present moment, without judgment. This can be achieved by focusing on the breath, physical

sensations, thoughts, or emotions. The goal of mindfulness is to increase self-awareness and improve emotional regulation.

3. How to practice: Meditation and mindfulness can be practiced in many different ways, including:

a. Sitting meditation: Sitting in a quiet, comfortable place, focusing on the breath or a specific object or sound.

b. Moving meditation: Incorporating mindfulness into physical movements, such as yoga or tai chi.

c. Mindful breathing: Focusing on the sensation of the breath moving in and out of the body.

d. Body scan: Lying down and focusing on the physical sensations in each part of the body, from head to toe.

4. Benefits: Meditation and mindfulness have been shown to have several health benefits, including:

a. Reduced stress and anxiety: By promoting relaxation and reducing feelings of stress and tension, meditation and mindfulness can help to reduce symptoms of stress and anxiety.

b. Improved sleep: Regular practice of meditation and mindfulness can improve sleep quality and reduce insomnia.

c. Increased self-awareness: By bringing attention to the present moment, meditation and mindfulness can help increase self-awareness and improve emotional regulation.

d. Enhanced cognitive function: Regular practice of meditation and mindfulness can improve cognitive function and increase focus and attention.

5. Precautions: Meditation and mindfulness are generally safe for most people, but it is important to check with a doctor before starting if you have any health conditions or mental health

                    Unleashing Your Inner Calm

concerns. Additionally, some people may experience feelings of anxiety or distress during meditation or mindfulness practices, especially if they have a history of trauma or mental health conditions. If this occurs, it is important to stop and seek medical advice.

Overall, meditation and mindfulness are powerful tools for reducing stress, improving well-being, and enhancing overall health and happiness. Whether practiced alone or as part of a group, these practices can help promote relaxation, increase self-awareness, and improve physical and mental functioning.

CHAPTER 3: MODIFYING LIFESTYLE HABITS

- Importance of sleep for a healthy nervous system

Sleep is important for a healthy nervous system because it allows the brain and body to rest, recharge, and perform essential functions that support physical and mental well-being.

1. Nervous system function: Sleep plays a critical role in the function of the nervous system, which includes the brain and the spinal cord. During sleep, the brain is able to process information, consolidate memories, and regulate mood and emotions. Additionally, the spinal cord is able to perform maintenance functions that help to keep it healthy and functioning properly.

2. Brain restoration: During sleep, the brain is able to perform essential restorative functions, including removing waste products and repairing damaged tissues. These functions help to maintain overall brain health and reduce the risk of neurodegenerative conditions such as Alzheimer's and Parkinson's.

3. Mental health: Sleep is also important for mental health, as it has been linked to reduced symptoms of depression, anxiety, and stress. In addition, adequate sleep can improve mood, increase emotional stability, and boost overall well-being.

4. Physical health: Sleep is essential for physical health as well, as it helps to regulate hormones, maintain a healthy immune system, and promote tissue growth and repair. Additionally, adequate sleep has been linked to a reduced risk of various health conditions, including heart disease, stroke, and type 2 diabetes.

5. Quality and quantity: The quality and quantity of sleep are both important for a healthy nervous system. Most adults need 7-9 hours of sleep each night, and the quality of sleep can be improved by creating a sleep-conducive environment, avoiding caffeine and alcohol, and practicing good sleep habits, such as maintaining a consistent sleep schedule.

Overall, sleep plays a critical role in the function of the nervous system and is essential for physical and mental well-being. Adequate sleep helps to promote brain restoration, improve mental health, and reduce the risk of various health conditions. By prioritizing sleep and creating a sleep-conducive environment, individuals can support their nervous system and overall health.

- The role of diet and exercise in reducing stress

Diet and exercise play an important role in reducing stress and maintaining overall physical and mental health.

1. Diet: A healthy diet rich in nutrients and antioxidants can help reduce stress and support overall health. Foods that are high in vitamins B, C, and E, such as leafy greens, fruits, and nuts, can help to reduce stress and improve mood. Additionally, omega-3 fatty acids found in foods like fatty fish, chia seeds, and flax seeds, can help to improve mood and reduce anxiety.

2. Exercise: Regular exercise has been shown to be an effective way to reduce stress and improve mental health. Exercise releases endorphins, which are natural mood-enhancers, and can also help to reduce feelings of anxiety and depression. Exercise can also improve sleep quality and reduce feelings of stress and tension in the body.

3. Combination of diet and exercise: A healthy diet and regular exercise can have a synergistic effect in reducing stress. A balanced diet that provides the necessary nutrients to support the body, combined with regular exercise, can help to reduce stress and promote overall physical and mental well-being.

4. Stress-reducing activities: In addition to diet and exercise, engaging in stress-reducing activities such as mindfulness, yoga, or deep breathing exercises, can also help to reduce stress and improve mental health.

Overall, a healthy diet and regular exercise can play an important role in reducing stress and promoting overall physical and mental health. By combining healthy habits with stress-reducing activities, individuals can support their nervous system and maintain overall well-being.

- Limiting caffeine and alcohol consumption

Limiting caffeine and alcohol consumption is important for maintaining a healthy nervous system and overall well-being.

1. Caffeine: Caffeine is a stimulant that can increase alertness and energy levels, but it can also cause negative effects on the nervous system. Caffeine can interfere with sleep, cause anxiety and jitters, and increase heart rate and blood pressure.

2. Alcohol: Alcohol is a central nervous system depressant that can have negative effects on mood and behavior. Chronic alcohol consumption can lead to long-term changes in the brain, and can result in impaired cognitive function, decreased motor skills, and a decreased ability to handle stress.

3. Recommended limits: It is recommended to limit caffeine consumption to no more than 400mg per day, which is equivalent to about 4 cups of coffee. Additionally, it is recommended to limit alcohol consumption to no more than one drink per day for women and two drinks per day for men.

4. Benefits of limiting consumption: Limiting caffeine and alcohol consumption can have numerous benefits for the nervous system, including improved sleep quality, reduced anxiety and stress, improved cognitive function, and reduced risk of long-term health problems.

Overall, limiting caffeine and alcohol consumption is important for maintaining a healthy nervous system and overall well-being. By following recommended limits, individuals can support their nervous system and reduce the risk of negative health effects.

CHAPTER 4: MANAGING STRESS

- Identifying sources of stress

Identifying sources of stress is an important step in managing stress and maintaining overall well-being.

1. Common sources of stress: There are many different sources of stress, including work, relationships, financial issues, and health problems. Stress can also result from major life changes, such as moving, starting a new job, or losing a loved one.

2. Personal stressors: It is important to identify personal stressors, which are unique to each individual. Personal stressors may include worries about health, relationships, or career, and can also include underlying mental health conditions such as anxiety or depression.

3. Triggers: Triggers are events or situations that cause a stress response. Identifying personal triggers can help individuals to better manage stress and avoid stressful situations when possible.

4. Stress journal: Keeping a stress journal can be an effective way to identify sources of stress and understand personal triggers. In a stress journal, individuals can write down when they feel stressed, what caused the stress, and how they coped with the stress.

5. Stress inventory: Taking a stress inventory can help individuals to identify sources of stress and understand the impact that stress is having on their lives. Stress inventories can be found online or through a mental health professional.

Overall, identifying sources of stress is an important step in managing stress and maintaining overall well-being. By understanding personal stressors and triggers, individuals can better manage stress and reduce the negative effects of stress on their lives.

- Using stress management techniques such as time management and goal-setting

Using stress management techniques, such as time management and goal-setting, can help individuals to reduce stress and improve overall well-being.

1. Time management: Effective time management can help individuals to prioritize tasks, avoid feeling overwhelmed, and reduce stress. Techniques such as creating to-do lists, prioritizing tasks, and avoiding procrastination can help individuals to manage time more effectively.

2. Goal-setting: Setting realistic and achievable goals can help individuals to stay focused and motivated, and can also reduce stress. When setting goals, it is important to consider both short-term and long-term goals and to break down larger goals into smaller, manageable tasks.

3. Prioritization: Prioritizing tasks and focusing on the most important tasks first can help individuals to avoid feeling overwhelmed and reduce stress. By focusing on the most important tasks first, individuals can avoid feeling like they are falling behind and can reduce stress.

4. Delegation: Delegating tasks to others can help individuals to reduce stress and avoid feeling overwhelmed. By delegating tasks to others, individuals can focus on the most important tasks and avoid feeling like they have too much to do.

5. Self-care: Taking time for self-care, such as exercise, meditation, and relaxation, can help individuals to reduce stress and improve overall well-being. By taking time for self-care, individuals can recharge and avoid feeling overwhelmed.

Overall, using stress management techniques such as time management and goal-setting can help individuals to reduce stress and improve overall well-being. By prioritizing tasks, delegating tasks to others, and taking time for self-care, individuals can better manage stress and maintain overall well-being.

- Seeking support from friends, family, or a therapist

Seeking support from friends, family, or a therapist can be an effective way to manage stress and improve overall well-being.

1. Support from friends and family: Talking to friends and family about stress and seeking support from them can help individuals to reduce stress and improve overall well-being. Having a supportive network of friends and family can help individuals to feel less isolated and can provide a source of comfort and support.

2. Professional support: A mental health professional, such as a therapist, can provide support and guidance for managing stress. A therapist can help individuals to identify sources of stress, develop coping strategies, and improve overall well-being.

3. Group therapy: Group therapy can provide a supportive environment for individuals to discuss stress and receive support from others who are also experiencing stress. Group therapy can also provide opportunities for individuals to learn coping strategies and develop a sense of community.

4. Online support: Online support groups and forums can provide individuals with a supportive community to discuss stress and receive support from others. Online support can be especially helpful for individuals who live in rural or remote areas, or for individuals who are unable to attend in-person support groups.

5. Hotlines and crisis lines: Hotlines and crisis lines can provide immediate support for individuals who are experiencing stress and need help. Hotlines and crisis lines can be a valuable resource for individuals who are in crisis or who are feeling overwhelmed.

                    Unleashing Your Inner Calm

Overall, seeking support from friends, family, or a therapist can be an effective way to manage stress and improve overall well-being. By seeking support and receiving help, individuals can better manage stress and maintain overall well-being.

Unleashing Your Inner Calm

CHAPTER 5: CULTIVATING RESILIENCE

- Building emotional intelligence and self-awareness

Building emotional intelligence and self-awareness can be an effective way to manage stress and improve overall well-being.

1. Emotional intelligence: Emotional intelligence refers to the ability to recognize and manage one's own emotions, as well as the emotions of others. By developing emotional intelligence, individuals can better understand and regulate their own emotions, which can help to reduce stress.

2. Self-awareness: Self-awareness refers to the ability to understand one's own emotions, thoughts, and behaviors. By increasing self-awareness, individuals can identify sources of stress and develop strategies for managing stress.

3. Mindfulness: Mindfulness is a technique for becoming more aware of the present moment and paying attention to one's thoughts, feelings, and surroundings. By practicing mindfulness, individuals can increase self-awareness and reduce stress.

4. Emotional regulation: Emotional regulation refers to the ability to manage one's emotions in a healthy and adaptive way. By developing emotional regulation skills, individuals can reduce stress and improve overall well-being.

5. Communication skills: Effective communication skills can help individuals to manage stress and improve overall well-being by reducing conflicts, improving relationships, and increasing emotional intelligence.

6. Stress management techniques: Techniques such as deep breathing, progressive muscle relaxation, and meditation can help individuals to increase emotional intelligence and self-awareness, and to reduce stress.

Overall, building emotional intelligence and self-awareness can be an effective way to manage stress and improve overall well-being. By developing emotional intelligence, self-awareness, and stress management skills, individuals can better understand and manage their emotions, reduce stress, and improve overall well-being.

- Practicing gratitude and positive thinking

Practicing gratitude and positive thinking can be an effective way to manage stress and improve overall well-being.

1. Gratitude: Gratitude involves focusing on the positive aspects of one's life and expressing appreciation for them. Practicing gratitude can help individuals to reduce stress and improve overall well-being by promoting a positive outlook and reducing negative thoughts.

2. Positive thinking: Positive thinking involves focusing on the positive aspects of situations and reframing negative thoughts. By practicing positive thinking, individuals can reduce stress and improve overall well-being by reducing negative thoughts and promoting a more optimistic outlook.

3. Journaling: Journaling can help individuals to practice gratitude and positive thinking by providing a space to reflect on the positive aspects of their lives and to express appreciation.

4. Affirmations: Affirmations are positive statements that individuals can repeat to themselves to promote positive thinking and reduce stress. By repeating affirmations, individuals can improve their self-esteem and reduce stress by focusing on positive thoughts and beliefs.

5. Mindfulness: Mindfulness is a technique for becoming more aware of the present moment and paying attention to one's thoughts, feelings, and surroundings. By practicing mindfulness, individuals can increase self-awareness and reduce stress.

Overall, practicing gratitude and positive thinking can be an effective way to manage stress and improve overall well-being. By focusing on the positive aspects of life, expressing gratitude, and reducing negative thoughts, individuals can reduce stress and improve overall well-being.

- Engaging in activities that bring joy and fulfillment

Engaging in activities that bring joy and fulfillment is an important aspect of stress management and overall well-being.

1. Hobbies: Engaging in hobbies and other leisure activities can bring joy and fulfillment, reducing stress and improving overall well-being.

2. Social activities: Spending time with friends and family and engaging in social activities can bring joy and fulfillment, reducing stress and improving overall well-being.

3. Exercise: Regular exercise can bring joy and fulfillment by providing an outlet for stress and improving overall health and well-being.

4. Volunteer work: Engaging in volunteer work and helping others can bring joy and fulfillment by providing a sense of purpose and improving overall well-being.

5. Creative pursuits: Engaging in creative pursuits such as art, music, and writing can bring joy and fulfillment, reducing stress and improving overall well-being.

Overall, engaging in activities that bring joy and fulfillment is an important aspect of stress management and overall well-being. By engaging in activities that bring happiness and a sense of purpose, individuals can reduce stress and improve overall well-being.

CHAPTER 6: MAINTAINING BALANCE

- Importance of finding balance in all aspects of life

Finding balance in all aspects of life is important for managing stress and improving overall well-being.

1. Work-life balance: Balancing work and personal life can help individuals to reduce stress and improve overall well-being by avoiding burnout and reducing feelings of overwhelm.

2. Physical health: Maintaining physical health through a balanced diet and regular exercise can reduce stress and improve overall well-being by promoting good health.

3. Emotional well-being: Balancing emotional well-being through self-care, therapy, and stress management techniques can reduce stress and improve overall well-being by promoting positive emotions.

4. Relationships: Balancing relationships with friends, family, and partners can reduce stress and improve overall well-being by promoting strong social connections.

5. Personal growth: Balancing personal growth through education, self-reflection, and other personal development activities can reduce stress and improve overall well-being by promoting self-awareness and personal growth.

Overall, finding balance in all aspects of life is important for managing stress and improving overall well-being. By prioritizing and balancing different aspects of life, individuals can reduce stress and improve overall well-being.

- Making time for self-care and relaxation

Making time for self-care and relaxation is important for managing stress and improving overall well-being.

1. Daily routines: Incorporating self-care activities into daily routines can help individuals to prioritize self-care and reduce stress.

2. Relaxation techniques: Engaging in relaxation techniques such as deep breathing, progressive muscle relaxation, and meditation can reduce stress and improve overall well-being.

3. Hobbies and leisure activities: Engaging in hobbies and other leisure activities can bring joy and fulfillment, reducing stress and improving overall well-being.

4. Sleep: Getting adequate sleep is an important aspect of self-care and can improve overall well-being by reducing stress and promoting good physical and mental health.

5. Regular breaks: Taking regular breaks from work or other demanding activities can help individuals to reduce stress and improve overall well-being by allowing for rest and relaxation.

Overall, making time for self-care and relaxation is important for managing stress and improving overall well-being. By prioritizing self-care and relaxation, individuals can reduce stress and improve overall well-being.

- Seeking professional help if needed.

Seeking professional help can be an important part of managing stress and improving overall well-being.

1. Therapy: Therapy can help individuals to identify and manage sources of stress, improve emotional well-being, and develop coping strategies.

2. Medical support: Medical support can be necessary for individuals with conditions such as anxiety, depression, and other mental health conditions that may be contributing to stress.

3. Support groups: Support groups can provide a safe and supportive environment for individuals to connect with others facing similar challenges and receive emotional support.

4. Medication: In some cases, medication may be necessary to manage symptoms of stress and improve overall well-being.

Overall, seeking professional help is an important aspect of managing stress and improving overall well-being. By seeking help from a therapist, medical professional, support group, or other resources, individuals can reduce stress and improve overall well-being. It is important to note that seeking professional help is not a sign of weakness, but rather a proactive step towards improved well-being.

CHAPTER SEVEN: FOODS THAT CAN BE USED TO CONTROL THE NERVEOUS SYSTEM

> **Complex Carbohydrates: Eating complex carbohydrates such as whole grains and vegetables can increase the production of serotonin, a neurotransmitter responsible for regulating mood and reducing stress.**

Complex carbohydrates play a role in controlling the nervous system by:

1. Providing energy: Complex carbohydrates are an important source of energy for the body and the brain, helping to regulate the nervous system by providing a steady supply of fuel.

2. Stabilizing blood sugar levels: Complex carbohydrates help to stabilize blood sugar levels, which can help to reduce symptoms of stress and anxiety by providing a stable source of energy.

3. Supporting brain function: Complex carbohydrates are important for brain function, as they are used by the brain to produce neurotransmitters, which help to regulate mood and reduce symptoms of stress and anxiety.

4. Promoting relaxation: Some complex carbohydrates, such as whole grains, contain magnesium, which is known to promote relaxation and reduce symptoms of stress and anxiety.

5. Reducing inflammation: Some complex carbohydrates, such as fiber-rich foods, can help to reduce inflammation in the body, which can reduce symptoms of stress and anxiety.

Consuming complex carbohydrates as part of a balanced diet can play a role in controlling the nervous system by providing a stable source of energy, supporting brain function, promoting relaxation, and reducing inflammation.

> **Omega-3 Fatty Acids: Foods's high in omega-3 fatty acids, such as salmon and walnuts, have been shown to positively affect brain function and can help reduce anxiety and depression.**

Omega-3 fatty acids play a role in controlling the nervous system by:

1. Supporting brain function: Omega-3 fatty acids are important for brain function and have been shown to support brain health and reduce symptoms of stress, anxiety, and depression.

2. Reducing inflammation: Omega-3 fatty acids have anti-inflammatory properties and can help to reduce inflammation in the body, which can reduce symptoms of stress and anxiety.

3. Regulating mood: Omega-3 fatty acids have been shown to regulate mood and improve symptoms of depression and anxiety.

4. Improving sleep quality: Omega-3 fatty acids have been shown to improve sleep quality, which can help to reduce symptoms of stress and anxiety.

5. Reducing oxidative stress: Omega-3 fatty acids can help to reduce oxidative stress, which can reduce symptoms of stress and anxiety by reducing the impact of free radicals on the body.

Consuming omega-3 fatty acids as part of a balanced diet can play a role in controlling the nervous system by supporting brain function, reducing inflammation, regulating mood, improving sleep quality, and reducing oxidative stress. Good sources of omega-3 fatty acids include fatty fish, such as salmon and sardines, and plant-based sources, such as chia seeds, flaxseeds, and walnuts.

> **B-Vitamins: B-vitamins, particularly B6 and B12, play a key role in the production of neurotransmitters and can help maintain cognitive function and mood. Foods rich in B-vitamins include poultry, fish, eggs, and whole grains.**

B-vitamins, particularly B6 and B12, can play a role in controlling the nervous system by:

1. Regulating mood: B-vitamins, particularly B6 and B12, are involved in the production of neurotransmitters, such as serotonin and dopamine, which play a role in regulating mood.

2. Reducing stress: B-vitamins, particularly B6, have been shown to help reduce symptoms of stress and anxiety.

3. Improving brain function: B-vitamins, particularly B12, have been shown to support brain function and improve cognitive performance.

4. Reducing fatigue: B-vitamins, particularly B12, have been shown to reduce symptoms of fatigue and improve energy levels.

5. Maintaining nerve health: B-vitamins, particularly B12, are important for maintaining nerve health and reducing symptoms of nerve damage.

Consuming B-vitamins as part of a balanced diet can play a role in controlling the nervous system by regulating mood, reducing stress, improving brain function, reducing fatigue, and maintaining nerve health. Good sources of B-vitamins include animal-based foods, such as meat, poultry, and dairy, and fortified plant-based foods, such as fortified cereals.

> **Probiotics: Probiotics, the healthy bacteria found in fermented foods such as yogurt and kefir, have been shown to positively impact the gut-brain axis and can help regulate the nervous system.**

Probiotics, or beneficial bacteria found in the gut, can be used to control the nervous system in several ways:

1. Regulating mood: Probiotics have been shown to impact the production of neurotransmitters in the gut, which can play a role in

   Unleashing Your Inner Calm

regulating mood and reducing symptoms of anxiety and depression.

2. Improving gut health: A healthy gut microbiome can have a positive impact on overall health and well-being, including reducing symptoms of stress and anxiety.

3. Reducing inflammation: Probiotics have been shown to reduce levels of inflammation in the body, which has been linked to a range of health problems, including stress and anxiety.

4. Enhancing immunity: Probiotics have been shown to enhance the immune system, which can play a role in reducing stress and anxiety.

5. Regulating cortisol levels: Cortisol is a hormone released in response to stress. Probiotics have been shown to regulate cortisol levels, reducing symptoms of stress and anxiety.

Consuming probiotics as part of a balanced diet or through supplements can play a role in controlling the nervous system by regulating mood, improving gut health, reducing inflammation, enhancing immunity, and regulating cortisol levels. Good sources of probiotics include fermented foods, such as yogurt, kefir, and sauerkraut, and probiotic supplements.

➢ **Hydration: Staying hydrated by drinking plenty of water is important for maintaining the proper function of the nervous system. Dehydration can lead to symptoms such as fatigue, headaches, and decreased cognitive function.**

Hydration can be used to control the nervous system in several ways:

1. Reducing fatigue: Staying hydrated can help reduce fatigue, which can impact mental and emotional well-being, and increase stress and anxiety levels.

2. Regulating body temperature: Hydration helps regulate body temperature, which is important for overall health and well-being, including reducing symptoms of stress and anxiety.

3. Improving cognitive function: Hydration has been shown to improve cognitive function, including attention and memory, which can play a role in reducing stress and anxiety levels.

4. Regulating mood: Dehydration has been linked to changes in mood, including feelings of irritability and anxiety. Staying hydrated can help regulate mood and reduce symptoms of stress and anxiety.

5. Reducing headaches: Dehydration is a common cause of headaches, which can increase symptoms of stress and anxiety. Drinking enough water can help reduce headaches and improve overall health and well-being.

Overall, staying hydrated by consuming enough water and other hydrating fluids, such as herbal teas and fruit-infused water, can play a role in controlling the nervous system by reducing fatigue, regulating body temperature, improving cognitive function, regulating mood, and reducing headaches. It is recommended to drink at least 8 glasses of water per day.